WEIGHT LOSS

...The Truth

Burn Fat, Build Muscle & Lose Weight....
Naturally!

What's inside

How to stop the process of storing fat!

Do aerobics do anything for me?

How hard should I exercise?

When will I see results, really!

What is CNS and how does it control my progress, or lack of it?

Why can't I lose weight?

How do I train my mind for results?

..............................Find out what it "really" takes!

Written By Former Bodybuilder
Bill Thomas

Distributed by
Bill Thomas
P.O.Box 70133
Staten Island NY 10307-1101

Copyright January 28, 2005
By Bill Thomas
P.O.Box 70133
Staten Island NY 10307-1101

ISBN-13: 978-1441474094
Manufactured in the United States of America

Liability Disclaimer

While the author has obtained the information contained in this book as the
result of personal experience as a weightlifter and former Bodybuilder, He
makes no implication of guaranteed results, as each individual is uniquely
different in physical condition and body type; the experience relayed and the
results may not be the same, any individual who decides to undertake any
type of exercise ,dieting or weight loss program does so at their own risk and
with prior consent from their Medical Doctor, The author will not, in any way
be held liable in the event of death or physical injury as a result of
information offered in this book.
This book is offered as a tool to help the reader better understand the process
of weight reduction and how the body tries to achieve that result.

Exercise & Diabetes
Insulin dependent diabetics should be aware of a condition known as *Lactic
Acidosis and consult a physician prior to any intense exercising routine.

 *Lactic acidosis is a condition caused by the buildup of lactic acid in the
body. It leads to acidification of the blood (acidosis) and is considered
potentially life threatening. Know the symptoms of Lactic Acidosis and
consult with your physician.

Preface

Let me first introduce myself, my name is William Thomas, I am the author and publisher of this personal experience book dealing with the issue of muscle development and weight loss, specifically, how to achieve it naturally, that is, without the use of sometimes dangerous diet supplements.

In the 23 plus years since my experience with resistance training I still find it hard to believe that a basic, concise, understandable and easy to read source of information, making clear the requirements necessary to truly achieve the goal of weight reduction is almost impossible to find. So I produced it.

The purpose of the book is to provide information on exercise and weight loss through a simple understanding of what the body requires to achieve the ultimate result of fat reduction, and remember, fat reduction is not as easy to obtain as "weight loss" which is usually water and protein mass (muscle) with very little fat reduction, if any at all.

I personally believe, and I think you do as well that weight loss has not been truly achieved unless there has been a significant amount of fat reduction with a reasonable amount of muscle development and an overall better general feeling of good health.

Along with regular exercise, proper diet and a naturally increased rate of your body's metabolism you should obtain the results that you want to obtain as I did.

This book will provide an understanding of **How to Train, What to Expect, Why it's Necessary, What Controls Your Progress or lack of it, When to Realistically Expect to See Results, and How Much Exercise Is Enough** to achieve that goal. Just a few of the highly important and often overlooked or least understood areas necessary to succeed.

My qualifications are based on my personal experience as a weight lifter and former Body builder, experiencing the effects of resistance training first hand and learning through feel and basic knowledge of physical development, that weight loss and muscle development were both occurring at the same time, and although building muscle required a significantly higher level of effort to achieve, the same physical changes were taking place, once I realized that certain "feelings" were normal and an indication that the change was taking place, I was able to achieve my goal, its this same understanding that will empower you, as well as the millions and millions of others who never truly understood what was happening during exercise enough to be successful in reaching that level of "stimulation" each and every single day that they make that effort.

Finally

I've decided to pass this experience and crucial understanding on by writing this book "Weight Loss.... The Truth. What It Really Takes to Lose Weight," making it available to anyone who may find interest in the subject or are simply tired of just treading the water at best.

During the past 20 plus years

It seems that truth and reality have been replaced with false hope, misrepresentation and fine print, which has led us all to truly believe that overindulging is perfectly fine because the next scientific breakthrough will be an even better "miracle" in a bottle at "just $29.95" and *that* will be the one that reverses the suddenly noticeable spiraling out of control weight gain problem; and, be the one that actually works!

It surprises me that so much of the public actually believe, and defend that belief, that all of these supplements are proven "safe" and in some way regulated by the FDA, therefore OK to mix and match with casual recklessness!
Not realizing that there may be consequences for altering their body's natural chemical balance and interfering with the production of critical enzymes that are naturally occurring and necessary in order to naturally increase metabolism and naturally burn fat efficiently,

not realizing that simply stopping the use of these supplements does not guarantee that the body will "instantly" restart its normal enzyme production functions....this can sometimes take weeks or even months to become stabilized, which is why we almost always regain any weight that we *may* have lost during that time of use, plus additional weight that we may never have even had in the first place during those weeks that follow!

This Is Why

Most of us just go back on the supplement again or find another one in an effort to regain some control, control which we never really had in the first place. Unfortunately we really don't know what else to do.

So we struggle and continue to gain weight!

Ironically

These are the same "vicious circle" effects that bodybuilders experience when taking steroids to alter *their* body's chemical and enzyme production process. Their system basically shuts down during use due to supplement overload.

The result is

When they "off cycle" they lose much of the muscle mass that they had packed on during use. For them, this loss in muscle mass and water occurs because the body's chemical producing organs such as the liver, thyroid and adrenaline gland aren't functioning properly anymore and since they were never capable of production equal to the previous levels obtained through the supplementation, it causes many steroid users to never really "*off cycle*" which is what increases *their* risk of physical injury and even death.

The body just doesn't like to be chemically altered!

Dieters don't alter their system quiet as much as a bodybuilder on steroids will, but the alteration still occurs and the results are basically the same. Diet supplements are not to be taken carelessly if taken at all and when they are used they should be taken as part of a strict diet and exercise program that should always be supported by your medical doctor. Diet supplements are drugs regardless of whether their chemical based or "all natural" herbs, Remember, everything ends up in the blood and gets processed by the kidneys and liver; so improperly used; even herbs can be extremely dangerous.

Unfortunately, so many people have been so misled for so long that they simply aren't aware of what the truth is anymore, worst yet is that we've created, (*because of our own belief in "science fiction"*) a generation of completely oblivious adolescents who are having real problems with just being too overweight and having nobody to turn to for help. They certainly can't turn to us because we led them down this road in the first place, but who knew, we took information for the face value of it and refused to pay any attention to the fine print, we refused to believe that we might be relying on misrepresentation and over exaggerated claims in most cases, sure it sounded real enough but that doesn't change the situation we're all in now.

The damage is done.

Sadly, sounding real enough doesn't help those who now resolve to trying anything and everything in an effort to find their own solution; mixing and matching dangerous concoctions of diet supplements and starvation dieting, possibly causing irreparable damage to themselves!

.

I cant stress enough the importance of medical permission prior to engaging in a diet and exercise program, exercise that forces REAL muscle stimulation and produces real results Prolonged physical stress, a healthful diet, a daily multivitamin, *a change in thinking*...and an apple; when the urge to eat something pops up out of nowhere at 9 o'clock at night is all it really takes!
Introduce this book to your family and friends, introduce this book to your group or organization, introduce this book to your company's health care and benefits officer,

introduce this book to your local school authority,
bring it to a PTA meeting just get it out there
and help make the needed change that we need
to make, everyone will benefit from something in
it.....I'm sure of it!

First of all, I want to congratulate you on the purchase of this
book. The first thing that many of you will do is look through
the pages searching for something that might pertain to your
specific need and jump right to it...DON'T

Because if you really knew what the problem was you
wouldn't be here reading this book... trust me!

It's important that you read the pages that follow in the order
that they're presented and that you read them often.

During the first 6 months you'll experience many changes and
your understanding of them will be found in these pages so
refer to them.

Regardless of your goals, whether they're to build solid
muscle for size and strength or reducing weight by burning the
stored fat that gets harder and harder to lose with every day
that goes by, you'll need to have a clear understanding of what
to expect from your future workouts as well as what will be
expected of you to be successful.

The information in this booklet is brief in explanation and
clearly understandable.

I'm confident you'll be happy with the results you *will* attain
and feel more comfortable with the pain and soreness you are
expected to achieve.

I encourage you to work hard, work out everyday, and never
lose sight of your ultimate goal no matter how great you may
begin to feel.

GOOD LUCK!

Here are a few important facts you should be aware of before you begin, we'll start off with the easy ones that some of us are already vaguely familiar with

1. Fat cannot be reduced simply by reducing caloric intake or taking a pill, it requires a little bit more effort than that. It's important that you accept one very important fact about the fat that our body's have stored and how your body regards it, your body will **never** turn to stored fat as a first option for a source of energy to perform every day functions when it's in need, It's just part of the human body's natural survival instinct, fat is just too difficult to break down and requires too much energy to process, and why should it try too, especially when there's a much easier source available to use.

    Meet the other source..... **Muscle**!

Pure protein & easily converted for energy.

Less muscle means that we get tired faster, we do less work and generally we sit around a lot more....gaining weight! Stopping the cycle is as simple as using the muscles we have and getting to know the muscles that we didn't even know we had. The human body is smart, it knows what muscles we're using; stops attacking them for energy and turns to the fat it so thoughtfully put aside for us, now, can you say "immediately" because it changes that fast, and in another section you'll find out why.

2. The muscles need constant stimulation to continue their resistance to the body's search for an easy energy source, once muscle stimulation stops we stop burning stored fat and begin to break down muscle tissue again, which is another reason why you'll NEVER look like a bodybuilder!!!....unless that's your objective and in that case then just keep working out with heavier and heavier weights and you'll reach that objective in a few years.

3. Physical training (mostly resistance exercise) raises the body's metabolism which dramatically alters how we process what we eat and burn stored fat deposits. A higher metabolism makes it easier to break down fat while preserving muscle for exercise.

4. Always remember that body weight should be reduced in a slow, steady and healthy manner. Rapid weight loss is usually little more than water and muscle mass, one of them you'll get back in a week or two (the water), the other is gone for good, that is unless we vigorously exercise to regain it (the muscle).

5. You should always workout to a mild sweat and then continue for another 30-45 minutes, sweating the entire time preferably. By the way, sweating does have a purpose, not only is it a natural cooling function during exercise but it flushes toxins from your body as well as being a great indicator to your level of effort. Sweating is a good thing, so sweat it!

6. Your body will constantly try to adjust to it's changing state of higher activity so without constantly pushing the muscles harder and harder in a slow and progressive manner we reach a performance plateau; that is, we stop burning fat, basically we change "modes" and start storing it again.

Why does this happen you ask?
It happens because the muscles that
we've using the most have become as
strong as they need to be, and if you
think about it for a second you'll
realize that you see people everyday
who have reached what I call a
"performance plateau" in their life;
it's why we see overweight physically
active people everyday, we know that
these people make an effort not to be
that way so how can it be possible, we
see it in the person who goes to the
gym all the time, expending no more
effort today than they did last week
but yet they don't seem to be losing
the pounds, they think there doing a
good thing, in fact they may even look
like they've gained weight, and they
probably have!

These people have simply become as strong
as **they** needed to be to get from one day to
the next, the body took over and decided it's
fine, and it went back to storing fat again.
This "change over" has been ignored since
the beginning of time, it's a natural
occurrence that we knew (as weight lifters)
we had to control in order to remain as lean
as possible, it's a change that **you** have to be

aware of to succeed. We'll find out how to avoid the change in another section, remember, your not in control of your body, something else is, and that you can control.

In regard to water consumption during a workout, always keep drinking to a minimum, after exercising water becomes more necessary for the obvious reasons as well as the not so obvious, water helps flush out the toxic chemicals formed in the body and muscles during a workout and during the recuperation process, the most obvious toxin that you'll soon get to know all too well will be lactic acid, this is the one that will be the cause of all the soreness you'll have, you'll feel it in about 2 days after you start making progress, ...if you do it right!

Breathing...sounds easy enough, right. You'd be surprised how many people do something so easy, so unbelievably wrong in the gym! Breathing properly means taking slow, deep and steady breathes while exercising, in weight training it means inhaling prior to a lift and releasing at the top of a lift, this helps regulate and control your pace of exercise and helps control your heart rate, it also strengthens your overall cardiovascular fitness, Breathing heavy and erratically is the wrong way to breathe, although unavoidable at first, still wrong. Think Control.

I strongly recommend the incorporation of free weights into whatever form of exercise routine you choose to perform, the added weight creates specific muscle stimulation which helps to increase the body's metabolism and speeds the fat burning process. Remember, stimulating your muscles into "irregular" activity is what gets the whole process of weight loss started.

SO HOW DO I START OUT!

Choosing the correct weight to use is not that easy to do, in fact a commonly made mistake is to start off using too much weight, which is what makes most people quit after the second or third day. Too much weight equals too much strain equals way too much pain afterwards!

First find a weight that you can lift or move about 35-40 times, rest for only 2 minutes at most, lift another 35-40 times and then stop, just perform the 2 sets at first until your muscles get used to the new activity,

This should be the "ideal weight" for that exercise. Remember, you won't find this ideal weight right away but in a few days you'll have it, just start off on the light side of the weight rack and you shouldn't have any problems.

Continue using this weight for at least 8 weeks As with anything new and especially weight training, everything will feel awkward in the beginning, you may feel as if your doing something wrong, in some way it won't feel like you think it should feel or it might feel awkward, it's normal and it's considered the adjustment phase. Your body will be trying to find the natural range of motion for the exercising your performing, your posture and body style. It's also the time when that "controller" I've been eluding to is finding out that "things are about to change!"

Just a word of caution here.

During first few weeks you may want to increase your "ideal weight" a little, because it's become "light" which is normal, however I would maintain the "35-40" rule though because you haven't developed a "structural foundation" yet, so take it slow at this early stage, nothing lasting was ever built on a weak foundation!.

The first month is pretty tough I agree, but that's when most people have decided that they don't want to try that hard to get what they really want and quit.

Your already ahead of any one of them because you have this information in your hand and because you'll know what to expect. The reality is this, it all gets a lot easier in about 6 weeks, plus your already going to start to see results!

A final note on the use of free weights by which I mean ankle weights, wrist weights, weighted belts, back packs, dumbbells, barbells, cable machines etc. It's anything that adds resistance to the muscles that your working, always remember to workout as hard as you feel you possibly can and you will see the improvements your looking for!

And don't be bashful, go out and buy a muscle related magazine sometime, the information you can get will be coming from people who obviously know what they're talking about!

The Importance Of Warm-Ups

Back in 1983 when I first drafted this booklet there were no scientific studies confirming the importance of warm-ups it was just something that those of us who were more seriously into working out knew about, and as I said earlier, we didn't talk very much about what we knew.

Today there are studies confirming it's benefits every where so I guess personal experience does account for something.

There are two types of warm-ups

Specific

General

Specific warm-ups would consist of stretching or bending a specific body part either weighted or not weighted at all. The intention is to loosen the muscle up in all of it's full range of motion so to reduce the risk of injury during exercise, it also "flushes" the muscle with fluid, this helps to eliminate the source of pain associated with your prior workouts, by flushing the muscle or group of muscles you remove the lactic acid build up which is a product that is created during muscle tissue replacement, tissue that has been replaced by new stronger muscle tissue while you've slept over the past two nights. These warm-ups and stretching exercises are especially helpful during the first few weeks when the most muscle cells are going to be destroyed and replaced by new stronger ones, this is when stiffness and soreness will be at it's worst

The stiffness you are likely experience will gradually be reduced during the next 6-8 weeks. During this time a number of good things are beginning to happen, for instance you should be starting to feel something called the "pump" and beginning to understand when it actually occurs and how to induce it.

We'll talk about that in a second.

General warm-ups consist of exercises that get many muscles moving at one time, this would be bicycling, walking or speed walking, running and swimming which is an excellent way to strengthen lower back muscles as well as the overall body in general.

As a general warm-up for most major upper body muscles including the arms, back, chest & abs I have used the push-up extensively, this can be done with so many variations in regard to hand placement going from a wide posture to a narrow one that it can actually become a great "specific" muscle group exercise i.e. shoulders, arms and pectorals.

For the lower body; walking, squatting and stretching will work well to loosen the muscles in the lower back, thighs & calves

For the record most aerobic exercising is nothing more than extended duration "warm-ups" so for this purpose they're perfect, however for the purpose of weight reduction they're not very effective because they fail to provide the muscle stimulation required to force the change!

He says, She says….
Who even knows any more?

The fact of the matter is that today, many people out there in the gym or at the supermarket just don't really know who's got the right answers when it comes to exercise, we all just trudge along and think that *we* have them until we discover that we're going backwards, or at the very least we're not losing as much as we thought we would be by now

I had someone tell me recently "everybody's different and we all have to find what works for us" but is that really true or is it just a common and easily acceptable excuse?

Well, just for those of us who aren't sure or think otherwise, it's an excuse and I'll explain why in a minute.

Here's where it all came from

Unfortunately, we get bombarded with uninformed opinions from "the friend" who feels great now that they hit the treadmill 5 days a week for a brisk "fast walk" but still have no real weight loss to talk about, or someone from the gym who isn't even there anymore because *they* weren't getting results that they expected to get, or maybe we just made our own assumptions based on the level of activity that we saw someone exhibiting on television in a commercial that was designed to sell us a new piece of exercise equipment which is practically "effortless" to use but is guaranteed to "trim your waist & hips in no time at all". Where ever it was that you stumbled across your information the bottom line is that we're led to think that it's supposed to be easy to do and if it wasn't effortless for *us* then it's just something that ....*doesn't work for our body*! Does that sound about right?

The fact is we simply have no idea what the real truth is anymore, and it's a perfect example of how little we actually know about our own body, specifically how it *really* works, *why* it stores fat, and what it takes to *reverse the process*, But even worst than that is that it's a perfect example of how brainwashed we've become by all this exaggerated hype in our desperate search for a simple & effortless solution to make it all just go away!...and it will, I promise
 But first let's get to the bottom of this "excuse" issue.
First of all, I think we can all agree that we're all human beings and our body's all

have the same enzyme producing internal organs right. So then we should also agree that when we consume food, our body's do exactly the same thing with that food that everyone else's body does with it, right. .....I can hear the "Thyroid" argument already, which is why you need to talk to your doctor before you do anything!

Now, back to class.

Our body breaks down food that we eat and the liver converts it into glucose for the fuel that we need in order to get us through the next few hours until we eat again; the excess calories are converted to glycogen that's stored away for later use, any excess glycogen is stored away attached to a fat cell, what's left is sent out of the body as waste. This is the information that we're all familiar with, basically, right, but why did we stop there? Why didn't we have any interest in the "conversion back to glucose and usage process?"

Its not that we **can't** convert this stored fat for use or that "my body doesn't want to burn fat" its knowing what it takes to *force* your body into burning fat!

Realize that your body functions on its own, you don't breathe because you say "breathe" you breathe because "your body" wants to breathe, *your body* wants to survive, that's its primary function and although you have master control capability you're really just along for the ride, do nothing to guide it, and it takes over.

Which is why we stored all this fat in the first place, it's our survival mode. Why does a bear store fat? They do it to get through the upcoming "emergency" of winter.

We store fat in case we have an upcoming emergency too, we're still evolving if you think about it, maybe in million years we'll stop this storage process and evolve to the full fledge "living in excess" mammals that we are, maybe!....maybe.

So now here we are back at the beginning again, what's right, and what do I have to do to get the results that seem to be so hard to get?

Remember, I said that the answer is simple so here it is.

Create a difference between the calories that you consume and the calories that you burn and you'll create the difference in your life that you want to create. STOP...I can hear it already..."We all know that" your saying ... and your right, the only real unknown here is "how much" we should be doing to create the change, how much "stimulation" does it take to trigger the fat burning process? The answer to that question is in the next chapter, but don't rush off just yet!...

Fat reduction is a direct result of effort *and* discipline, and as long as you really want it then there's no reason that you can't have it, resistance exercising is the most effective way to burn fat for several reasons.

First, resistance training stimulates our *central nervous system* and causes physical stress, this is the "good" stress, this stress triggers the body to release enzymes that speed up the metabolism "naturally" and increases the body's fat burning efficiency. Resistance training causes you to sweat in an effort to cool itself down, think of it as a high speed central air conditioning system for your body, burning calories about as fast as your real air conditioning system burns electricity. Resistance training causes you to work harder by requiring more effort necessary to do the work, and that burns calories

Resistance training preserves and builds muscle which creates a tremendous amount of physical stress on the body and again, physical stress burns tons of calories

Resistance training simply burns more fat than any other form of exercising there is because it simply requires more effort to perform, period.

What is resistance training?

Resistance training is any form of exercise that has resistance to it. It can be gravitational resistance as in weight lifting or mechanical resistance as in hydraulic pistons.

It's the force that causes you to work!

Remember, it's not supposed to be easy, *easy,* is what you can get away with when you've already achieved your goal, **maintenance** is what you get from "easy"... 3 days a week, 20 minutes a day is easy and it's great for a *maintenance program*, but..... not weight loss.

WHAT IS EXERCISE?

Many people think that exercise is doing something that some of us consider "not really exercise" but as long as we can get away with it then we say to ourselves "I went to the gym and worked out today."

We've been led to believe that exercise is what we're doing when we get on a treadmill or a stationary bicycle for 45 mins. a day. The fact is that exercise isn't supposed to be what we want it to be because then it would be easy wouldn't it. Exercise is not supposed to be an extension of our daily workload with the only difference being that we're doing it in a different atmosphere. Our body isn't *tricked* into burning off fat just because we're in a gym; it reacts to *what we do and how hard we make it work to get it done*!

Realize what we want to achieve, what it is that we want our bodies to do.

We want it to do more than just burn calories, we want it to burn stored fat, a hard process to undertake, and to do that we need to <u>make</u> it burn fat!

Exercise is *supposed* to be physically demanding, its *supposed* to be harder than anything else that we've done all day long, its *supposed* to stimulate the adrenal gland which in turn triggers chemical and physical reactions to occur that cause the body to require more fuel than you consumed at your last meal, exercise is *supposed* to burn fat but only if done to the necessary level of physical exertion that starts the whole process in motion.

Exercise is work!

When we exceed physical activity above what we know as *normal*, we start a process that most people don't realize they've started, I look at it as similar to a runaway train speeding down a hill, remember, you're just along for the ride.
Here's why:
Just because we've stopped exercising our body hasn't finished requiring fuel, the CNS took over long before you quit and is still sending signals to the muscles that they need to become stronger if their going to have to go through this again, this required the brain to stimulate the 'manufacturing" process and start building stronger muscle tissue, this also triggered the liver to produce enzymes that break down fat and allow it to be converted back to the fuel source we need for everything to keep going, realize that at

this point after exercising your motor is still in high gear, you might notice a slight sensation of "vibrating" or an internal trembling after exercising at one point, its normal.
Then, there's the actual repair process that's going on which continues for the next 48 hours day and night, and its all happening at the same time ....So your body is working *very* hard while your sitting back right now!

 The best part of it is that the body gets more efficient at burning fat as it becomes leaner and healthier.
Read that again!

The Pump

The "pump" as some like to call it is actually
a difficult feeling to describe, however as you
approach the moment during your workout
when it occurs and your not familiar with it
then you may never push for that extra 10%
to achieve it, it's a feeling of internal
explosion within the target muscle or group
of muscles, it's the point at which your
muscles approach that level of "peak density"
it's a feeling that most people would think
could be a "bad" feeling which is why so
many never reach it, it's here that body
language and focused concentration becomes
so important, where knowing what the
difference is between physical pain and
emotional pain, the point where your muscle
actually feels as if it's about to burst, and
you let it, sort of....and this isthe time that
you realize that your muscles have had a
"second gear" all along but were never
pushed hard enough to find it, and now, as
you squeeze out a few more reps your
thinking, ... that was incredible, it was better
than incredible, I never knew I could do that,
you feel like you just pushed over a
mountain, and then, ...with a blast of

adrenaline, you've become hooked on it, you've become hooked on the "feeling" of the acheivement of the "pump" explosion and its that feeling of achieving it, knocking down the wall you never knew could be knocked down, is what will bring you back tomorrow and everyday after that. It's the feeling that you will strive for and not finish your workout until you feel again.

That's "The Pump" and some where in your second month of weight training you'll find it!...Be ready!

The Central Nervous System
It controls everything.

Unfortunately, even today very few people taking up physical fitness, and that includes both the beginners as well as the advanced ranks realize that the CNS is actually what controls all of their gains and losses, for the ones looking to get muscular, some turn to steroids because they just don't know why the progress suddenly stopped, and they don't know what else to do. For the dieters looking to loose another 10 pounds they turn to OTC diet pills for the same reason, ...the progress suddenly just stopped, and they don't understand why.

So what happened?

Everyone will experience rapid improvements during the first 2-4 months, and you should be very happy with those results, confidence and self esteem are running through the roof, for both men and women and every thing seems to be almost perfect except... you may find yourself not progressing as much as you were only a few short weeks ago, but why... your doing the same quality work as you always have, ...so what's going on here?

Welcome to another natural phase that some people call "The Slump" no matter what *you* call it, when it happens it can be pretty bad, suddenly your loosing control of the grip you had on this thing, you try everything you can think of but you just cant figure it out, in fact you're starting to wonder if this is as good as it gets for you, is this as far as you can go? It's a bad feeling for most of us and at some point you'll have it too.

It can be such a frustrating feeling that many people actually give up and quit....*Don't do it*!

The reason for this slow down in progress is due to the CNS ability to adapt to "present" conditions, It's comfortable here where it is, just like when you were a couch potato and you gained the weight or when you were skinny and didn't have any muscle at all it was comfortable there, the answer is really simple if you think about it for a minute...what brought on all the progress in the first place? It was the change you made from your previous lifestyle!

Over the past few months, usually around 6th or 7th, your Central Nervous System

(CNS) has slowly gotten used to the new workload you've thrown at it....Remember the "Performance Plateau"

Try to remember that your body does things that we didn't tell it to do; it really does work on its own, don't forget that! It's going to try to tell you when its done enough work or reached a level of comfortable capacity, the CNS (central nervous system) has stopped sending messages to the brain for all that adrenalin that's helped you get this far, as far as your body's concerned, nothing else has changed and so **nothing further <u>has</u> to change**!

I personally went on for months before I realized the problem.

And here it is— It was the routine!

If your like most people you have developed a routine which is what your supposed to do, for example you probably go to the gym or work out the same time everyday, the same days every week, the same number of repetitions/sets, right down to the same positions and the same range of movement and so on. That's a lot of the "same old stuff" going on here!

Here's a slight contradiction, as important as routine was in getting you this far, it's what getting in your way now!

So, add some variety to your workouts from time to time by doubling up on one or two sets or adding a new exercise to the routine altogether, also ask yourself, are you doing the exercises in the strict form that they're supposed to be done? Can they be performed a little more cleanly? You'll be surprised how much of a difference this can make in the feel of a weight and how the changed movement effects the required level of exertion needed to do it.

Be creative, do something that creates real muscle stimulation and jolts the CNS again, don't let yourself get comfortable unless you want to stop progressing.

This is a good time to mention something that I read in the dictionary a long time ago and it made a huge difference in how I worked out ever since.

I looked up the definition of "strength" and it said that strength was *"the ability to manipulate weight"*

That was it, and that changed it all for me, that was how I learned how to get out of the "slump." I realized that the routine that I had developed was just that "routine" and even though I felt that I had become stronger and leaner I wasn't "strong" and I wouldn't be until I could "manipulate" the weight rather than just lift it, once I learned that, I started to make progress, becoming even leaner and burning fat again, since it was my goal to also become stronger, I did, your goal is to burn fat and lose weight and you will!

The amazing thing today is that most people aren't even aware of this stuff, but that's why steroid use is up 900% since 1980 and the diet planning industry expoldes every few weeks with a new "breakthrough" diet pill ..(and behind it all there's a bunch of monkeys living it up in the south pacific somewhere!)....laughing at all of us!

Bottom Line Is This....

Weight reduction requires muscle stimulation which causes CNS stimulation and the only way to achieve the two is through exerting our muscles beyond their normal "comfortable capacity" just a little bit more every few weeks, and remember it's the "extra effort" that we put into it that makes the difference between success and failure!....

As you may be starting to realize, there's so much more to exercising and exercising correctly for the desired benefit then just jumping on a treadmill for an hour a day and expecting noticeable results.

Your body does what you let it do, but its up to you to make it do what you want it to do!

Rest & Recuperation

I can't stress enough the importance of proper rest if you're going to achieve your ultimate goal of weight reduction.

We have all heard that the body needs time to recuperate from strenuous activity, well here's a news flash, it's true! Without sufficient recuperation time which is a full 48 hrs. after the last time you were at the gym or in your basement, your newly forming muscle cells would never heal and harden in time to sustain your next workout, which means, your body would be constantly replacing muscle cells that won't be as strong as the ones that you just destroyed during exercise. The eventual result of this would be a muscle that continues to weaken until it has become so exhausted that it fails completely and injury occurs. Here's a suggestion; avoid an injury!

Recuperation simply means that the muscle should not be "directly" worked for the recommended 48 hrs so that healing of the muscle tissue has been able to be completed, however normal day to day activities can be performed no matter how strenuous they may be because this is already considered a "normal" daily activity for your body. Remember, your body is already used to the work that it does every single day, whether its sitting on a couch or climbing a mountain, it's only the added physical activities that it has to recuperate from.

Rest

Is simply this .....sleeping.....8 hrs a day!

Get it and that's all that the body requires to perform this incredibly complex job of healing. Don't get it and again we're back to the injury issue.

Try to understand everything that the human body has to do just to keep up with your day to day activities and you'll *want* to get 8 hrs of sleep every night, your body just can't spare the tremendous amount of energy it would need to heal from strenuous exercise during the busy day, there's too much for it to do already, and make no mistake about it, strenuous resistance exercise results in massive muscular injury on a low level scale, but massive because its on the scale of large portions of the body's muscular mass, think about it in this way and you can see how hard it would be to find the energy required to make the repairs on that scale while at the same time trying to keep everything else working flawlessly on anything less than 8 hrs of sleep a night, the fact is that during the day you're a machine running at 100% all the time regardless of whether or not you're a couch potato or a soccer mom or dad. Your body is working at near capacity based on the activity level that it's been accustomed to, and there's a lot more going on than what we see on the surface, how about all the work that it does that we don't even think about, I'll just mention a few to give you a picture.

How about that bruise on your arm or leg that you don't even know how you ended up with, that's damaged tissue that it has to repair, or the several hundred viral encounters that it came across during your "usual" day out there in the world. Do I have to remind you that it's also responsible for keeping all of our internal organs functioning properly like your heart, lungs, liver, kidneys, and brain! I think that the picture is a little clearer now, if you think about it for a minute you'll realize that your body is under constant attack and is always hard at work.

It's those 8 hrs of sleep at night when everything in the body slows down enough to just "survive" it's during that time of "rest" that it devotes all of its energy to recover, destroy, and repair all that's wrong with it, considering all the work that it does during the day when we're awake, 8 hrs. hardly seems even close to enough but your body knows what knows needs to be fixxed and it gets to it, all it needs is the chance to do it!

So don't underestimate the value of sleep, for proper function, both physically and metabolically we need it.

Visualization

As you're beginning to realize more and more from the information your getting in this booklet, the mind and body are pretty powerful, so there's no reason to stop seeing the possibilities now, right!

The mind is a very powerful tool if you know how to make it work for you, you may have heard at some time that "what can be conceived can be created."

I learned this a very long time ago and it's true. To develop a realistic attitude in respect to your goals you have to understand the manner in which you pursue your goal and together they'll determine whether or not you'll achieve that goal. If you keep applying yourself in a manner that's proven unproductive in the past then you'll foster a negative attitude and never succeed.

Think Positive

Before you take on anything new in your life you have to first believe in yourself, look back at what you've accomplished in the past and realize that it's possible to improve and become better. For those who find it difficult to see yourself in your own mind as the

person that you want to be then THIS IS
VERY IMPORTANT.

If necessary, stand in front of a mirror and
close your eyes, every few seconds open and
"look yourself in the eye" when your doing
this "visualization" re-programing. But
preferably try to see yourself in your minds
eye so that you get used technique.

**What you want to do is get a true image of
yourself as you are now, then close your
eyes and, in your mind...**

begin changing how you see yourself until
you have re-shaped every part of your body,
.... until you can see the person you want
to see, then, get used to seeing that image in
your mind and look at it often, ...when your
in the gym look at the mirror and "see" the
other you, "see" your arms leaner, "see" your
legs thinner, see your hips narrower, see
your chest larger, and don't pass one without
"seeing" yourself in some way changing.
Always think of yourself in the body that you
really want, but be realistic and remember
that the body you have now is NOT the one
your comfortable with.

What you're actually doing with this process
is changing your present line of thought
from "what is" to "what will be," and

eventually this new thinking as well as your new image will become normal and natural in your mind, its called reprogramming your "inside mind" or your subconscious mind to think that what <u>it</u> can see is the new reality. It's the new image that you'll work towards from now on and every day whether its in the gym or at home, you'll see two images, the one that's real and the one that's going to be real, and remember this, no matter how different they are from each other it doesn't matter, because your mind will believe what you convince it to believe.

Now I'm sure that there are some people out there who are probably thinking " that doesn't work, I do that every day" but....*do you really?... and if you do, is it possible that your fostering a <u>negative</u> image by starting off with a negative "thought"?*
I want you to be open to the real power of visualization. How many times I have tested it is beyond a number, in fact there are studies on this as well now, which wasnt the case when I first wrote this stuff.

HERES HOW I LEARNED ABOUT THIS

A long time ago when I was trying to change my physical appearance just as you may be today, I went to the gym a lot, I would do a ton of exercises, In fact I would go there saying to myself that today I would do this, this, this and this, I'd even have a set number of reps and sets that I would do for each exercise right down to the weight that I would use in each one, I'd even think about it during the day and that was fine, in fact it's exactly what you have to do, mentally prepare yourself. So anyway, I'd go to the gym and I did everything that I said I would do right down to the last rep!

After a while I realized there was a problem, I got to a point where I knew that I must be getting stronger, I mean, I've been doing this with the same weight for a while now but I could only do the number of reps that I had "planned" to do, not realizing that I had built a barrier for myself that I couldn't get passed, in fact to make matters worst, in between sets I would just rest long enough to "see" myself doing that next, pre determined number of reps, one at a time, when I finished visualizing the set I would get back to the exercise and do "just that number that I saw myself do in my visualization" and not a single one more, because I couldn't!

So one day I decided that during my rest period I would add 4 more reps to the visualization that I was doing, and from the

very next set I was doing the 4 extra reps, they were harder to do, you better believe it, but in my mind I knew they would be, and just as hard as they were to do in my mind is just how hard they actually were to do on the bench, but the point was that I did them, so I learned something else that day.
Visualization works...... so believe in it!

As you might imagine I had to put it to the test just about anytime that I could for a while and with just about everything I came up with it worked the same way, If I thought that I can only run to the end of the block then that's as far as I'm going to get before I <u>decide</u> that it's time to start walking, if I say that I can't do it then I won't be able to and if I say that I can then I will.

In 2001, not realizing I was setting myself up for something to happen in the future, my father had said "why don't I quit smoking", I'd been smoking for over 27 years and tried to quit at least 6 times, I tried it all, but nothing ever lasted for very long. So I just said "I think I will, in fact I'm going to quit on my birthday" which was 3 months away at that time, now for the next 3 months, and not cutting back at all, I wouldn't even think about that day, and then it came, 3 months had gone by already. I put down the pack and without any resistance or the slightest hesitation, put on a patch and I quit....that was in 2001 and I never looked back ...ever!

That happened because I visualized it happening. I trained my mind to accept that I would be a non-smoker on that day, and I was.
Just think it and then do it, if you can see it then you can acheive it! Believe it!

Exercise & Muscle Failure

I think that we all know by now that strenuous exercise should consist of a series of movements that will cause the muscles to become so fatigued that they can't work anymore, if we don't know it or we're choosing to deny it, so...either know it now, or "accept" that your denying it, and accept the reality.

When we exercise, the idea is to push the muscles to the point of fatigue and eventually to straddle that fine line of muscle failure necessary to continually progress forward. By pushing the muscles to this point it will cause the central nervous system to react in several ways, first by releasing adrenaline, increasing metabolism and releasing growth hormone starting the cycle of breaking down, replacing and changing. Growth hormone is the valuable trigger that starts the whole "renew" process going, it gets its message from the CNS and it goes to work providing the material needed to replace the older, weaker muscle cells that you have just torn apart with new, stronger muscle cells that will be capable of withstanding this new workload you have just thrown at them, remember the part where, building muscle increases metabolism, well its during this rebuilding process that the body is burning up fuel at a high rate of consumption and getting the energy needed to do so from its only abundantly available sources it has left to use, the stored fat!

So the importance of exercising to the point of muscle exertion can not be stressed enough, without it you simply won't trigger the process to burn fuel and utilize fat stored in the body which is what its all about!

So now that you've accepted to achieve full muscle exertion, you wake up one morning and you hurt so bad that you can't even put on your socks! ...ouch

Well it is very likely that you may have, and I emphasize the word "may" have over trained just a little bit. Remember that sore is a good thing, because it say's that you went far enough to start making changes, but being immobile isn't such a good thing.

*** *Which brings to mind again the need to check with your physician to sign off on your ability to perform strenuous exercise, if you haven't done it yet then put down this booklet and check with*

your doctor, I can't stress enough how important that is!
OK ...

As far as the soreness and pain go, stretch it, move it go back to the warm-ups chapter and work it out, it'll get better and I can assure you that you'll be ready to get to the gym again in 2-3 days, still in some pain naturally but after your first exercise or set it'll all disappear like it was never even there. Knowing that alone and getting past it, again is what so many people never find out because they quit and never come back, ...SO DON'T QIUT NOW!

Also keep in mind how much of a confidence builder this alone will be, knowing that you just got past something that has stopped so many others, your self esteem is going to take off, overall you'll be feeling pretty good, in fact, I'll even go out on a limb here and say that you might even like the feeling, <u>pain and all!</u>

I should mention this although it may seem hard to believe right now, the pain and soreness will actually become "enjoyable" to you. It will become something that you will want to achieve each and every time that you exercise.

Ever heard the phrase "No Pain, No Gain" Well it has true meaning. The simple fact is that if you aren't getting sore then you have not caused your body and muscles to achieve failure, in other words, you haven't made any changes for that day, and, that's not your goal!

Note: It's especially important to remind you that during the first 3-6 months of training you should concentrate on fully developing and strengthening your new muscle growth before attempting to add more weight (resistance) to your routine, adding weight in the beginning can increase the possibility for muscle injury which can take a very long time to heal, muscle injury can be extremely painful and should be avoided if possible

Take things slow at first, it's important to "feel" your body ; feel what it's telling you, it's talking all the time and in the gym is the worst place to stop listening to it. It's body language and with a little time you'll know exactly how to listen to it, always remember that the line between constant progress and painful injury is a thin one!

You'll probably pick up on the body language in the first 4-8 weeks, so be expecting to notice it.

Forced reps
(An Advanced Muscle Building Technique)

This is an advanced form of training that will produce the muscular results that some of you may be looking for, however I strongly advise against this type of training until at least you have completed 8-10 months of weight resistance training on a 5-6 day per week routine. This type of training can cause muscular injury if a strong muscular foundation has not been sufficiently established. It is also a tecnique that will develop the "pump" as discussed in an earlier section, this technique can be used to simply get to the "next level" as needed from time to time and also to go well beyond anyplace that most people will ever need to go.

Although a common training method among experienced weight lifters and widely practiced, Forced reps are very similar to cheating movements during an exercise, first the exercise must be performed in the strictest manner and with complete control, I refer back the definition of strength, "it is the ability to manipulate weight" the ability to manipulate the weight you are using in order to perform strict, controlled movement.

Once you have mastered that discipline and control then you can experiment with forced reps!

A forced rep is a repetition that is "cheated" <u>after muscle failure</u>, that is, having used every bit of energy you have left you should be unable to perform another full repetition in strict manner, then, using a slight "jerking" motion or in some cases using the assistance of a "spotter" continue to lift or move the weight as many more times as possible, every additional rep builds pure muscle by aggressively stimulating the CNS and causing an added rush of adrenaline and signaling for the release of larger amounts of growth hormone resulting in massive gains in a very short period of time.

This type of weight training should not be continued for any extended period of time because of its aggressive nature alone, again this is NOT a beginners technique for training. Referring back to the "fine line between constant gains and painful injury" those interested in this type of muscle development will straddle this line every single day to obtain their goal.

Exercise and weight loss
Who's kidding who?

Weight loss as you no doubt have come to realize requires hard and thoughtful, persistent work and a brisk stroll through the park or on a treadmill isn't going to do it, although some may justify this thinking by asking " have you ever seen an overweight marathon runner before" in which I'd personally have to reply, no! Then again I'm sure that most people don't run 26 miles on a treadmill, every single day either. Besides I don't think that running is the only form of exercising that they do to stay in shape anyway.

Weight loss requires strenuous exercise, hard work, resistance training, reduced calorie diets, and proper rest for recuperation.

4 out of the 5 won't do it, it takes all 5 together to get to our goal.

One more thing, 20 minutes a day 3 days a week isn't even close to enough.....sorry.

It should be clear by now that when we engage in a strenuous exercise program there is usually a decrease in body fat content and a maintenance of lean body weight (muscle mass). The reason for this is simple, the body will not break down muscle for an energy supply in a time of need when those muscles are being used, only during this time of "active use" will the body engage in the much harder process of breaking down our stored fat supply, which is the goal here. For noticeable weight loss to be "real", strenuous exercise must be performed for 12-16 weeks at a minimum frequency of 5-6 days a week, ...5 days per week would be optimal. The training intensity should be performed to correspond to a minimum of 60% (but preferably 70%) of maximum pulse rate, or approximately 110-120 beats per minute, (not to exceed 85%...approx. 135 bpm) for most adults this should be your target heart rate for maximum benefit overall.

You should consult your physician to establish your specific recommended heart rate as overall physical condition will be an important consideration.

Anyone who has been on a crash diet knows that it's very easy to reduce body weight by as much as 5-10 pounds in a very short period of time, even in as little as 3 - 6 days. This reducing effect may be even more pronounced during starvation or semi-starvation diets. While these crash diets can provide a quick fix their unfortunate reality is that 75% of the weight loss is water and the rest is protein or muscle mass, there is little loss of body fat at all, not to mention the health danger associated with that type of dieting.

A rapid loss in body weight is counter productive if the ultimate goal is to change the body composition by reducing fat and increasing —or at least maintaining— the muscle mass. Again when a large amount weight loss is the goal, the key is to reduce body weight at a slow and steady rate of not more than 2-3 pounds per week over a longer space of time.

HOWEVER, that said, extreme dieting can be beneficial if only maintained for a short period of time usually no more than 30 days and done thoughtfully. This can jump start a process but should only be considered if exercising on a daily basis, I strongly recommend vitamins during this risky, but possibly effective approach.

Exercise and Diet

As important as exercise is, diet plays an even more important role in weight loss and body composition changes. The two important dietary factors are still the number of calories, and what kind. While it's hard for so many people to believe, there is rarely the need for any normal adult to consume less than 1000 calories for a woman and 1200 calories for a man to achieve adequate weight loss. In fact, most adults can lose weight on 1200-1400 calories per day

Here's something that you'll find hard to believe today. It's been known, for example that diets that do not contain an adequate supply of carbohydrates will not result in noticeable fat loss. In other words, to burn fat the body needs carbohydrates. If carbohydrates are not included in the diet during weight loss, then extra amounts of protein will be lost, instead of only the fat. The net effect of not having carbohydrates in your diet is the reduction of lean body weight, rather than body fat.

The ideal diet during weight loss that will achieve the best body composition results would be 50-60% of the total calories as complex carbohydrates (starches, whole grains, bread and vegetables), 20% as fat and 20% as protein.

For example, a 1200 calorie per day diet, a person would consume 660 calories (165 grams) of complex carbohydrates, 240 calories (27 grams) of fat and 240 calories (60 grams) of protein.

Some Key Points

To alter the overall body composition, it's necessary to participate in large muscle exercises. Recreational sports like golf, racquetball or swimming do not provide the adequate levels of muscular stimulation required to alter the fat/muscle ratio.

Regular resistance training that uses free weights. Cam devises, weight machines, hydraulics and cable devices, are necessary for preserving muscle mass during weight loss.

Calorie reduction should be accompanied with regular vigorous physical activity.

Rapid weight loss is usually due to water and muscle loss, with little fat reduction at all.

Never miss a day that you are expected to exercise, this helps establish discipline

Always keep a written log containing your exercise, day, date, time rep/set.

Always try to work out to a sweat

Visualize yourself in the gym or exercising throughout the day, and use visualization during exercise.

Remember that it will take approximately 3 months before you will begin to make permanent changes to your body's composition. Take your time, and don't rush.

As you begin, always start out slow and light, use weights that you can only lift or move 35-40 times for a total of 1-2 sets, increasing sets gradually resting no more than 2 minutes between sets at first.

Every now and then, perform your exercise differently in some way. Remembering to constantly stimulate the Central Nervous System.

The best time to exercise is after you have been active for at least several hours, usually in the early evening.

A good indication that the CNS has been highly stimulated will be a slight trembling soon after exercising. This is a normal condition and usually only accompanies extreme physical stress.

Routine is important, but when all else fails, change the routine.

Always concentrate on what your doing while exercising, think about your breathing, your movement and how honest your being with yourself in performing the exercise.

Heavy weights that can only be lifted a few times build muscle mass and strength. Lighter weights lifted more often (higher reps/sets) Burn more calories, build strength, endurance and physical definition.

Always build a solid foundation before attempting any experimental heavy lifts.

Lastly, you should consult your physician before beginning any strenuous weight training regime. I hope that you achieve your goals!

Juices for Weight Gain, Weight Loss & Energy

In each individuals own way, in our attempt to reach our goals we must learn how to eat properly.

This means knowing what kind of protein to eat and when to eat it, It means knowing how to load up on carbs prior to a workout. It often means using a blender or a juicer to prepare natural, healthy juice drinks specifically geared to the mix of nutrients you need to reach your desired goals.

For a weight gain drink this often means higher calorie foods, plus abundant carbohydrates and protein. For weight loss, you want to eliminate the high calorie foods but keep some of the high quality protein and natural carbohydrates for energy needs. You also want a good supply of fluids and plenty of vitamins and minerals. For high energy, a high proportion of natural carbohydrates is a smart choice.

In this section we'll take a look at how we can use juices to help reach our goals—and fast!

With a blender or juicer you can prepare the perfect meal in –a-glass to feed you body what it needs to cut the fat and keep the muscle, The weight loss drinks listed here in this section provide many healthy benefits including :

Adequate protein to prevent your body from having to burn it's own lean muscle tissue to provide itself with body energy

Adequate fluids to help prevent dehydration.

Vitamins and minerals (including electrolytes such as potassium) to help prevent deficiencies.

Carbohydrates for natural energy

Little or no fat

Low calorie doesn't mean low nutrition when it comes to natural juice drinks that you can easily make yourself

Juicing is one of the fastest and most healthful ways of getting energy building carbohydrates into your system. The juices in this category make excellent pre-workout energy boosters. Among the many benefits these energy drinks are:

Easily digestible

Quick, available energy

Contain complex and simple carbohydrates

B-vitamin energy "jump-starters"

We've all heard so much about carbohydrates in the last few years, But what are they?

Carbohydrates are complex chains of natural sugars that enter the blood stream as glucose, the simplest form of sugar.

The liver stores two thirds of this glucose as glycogen and supplies it to the body as energy is needed. Your body also stores glucose in your muscles as glycogen, it's also your muscles primary fuel.

Juice Drinks for Weight Gain

These special drinks for weight gain may be taken in addition to your regular meals. For rapid weight gain, they may be taken 3-times a day after breakfast, lunch and supper (or just before bedtime). The "Monster Gainer" for example, supplies more than 600 calories per drink to help gain pound after pound of solid muscle when you combine it with your weight training routine.

Fruit Blast

2 tbsp. All vegetable high quality protein powder

1/2 cup fresh melon

1/2 cup fresh strawberries

1/2 cup fresh papaya

Crushed ice

Super Gainer

4 tbsp. All vegetable high quality protein powder

2 cups whole milk

1 fresh orange

1/2 cup blueberries

1/2 cup raspberries

1/2 cup raw pecans or walnuts

Monster Gainer

3 heaping tbsp. All vegetable high quality protein powder

2 cups whole milk

1 cup coconut milk or coconut shred (both is better)

1 tbsp. honey

1 cup natural vanilla or Pistachio ice cream

Raw Power Gainer

3 heaping tbsp. All vegetable high quality protein powder

2 cups whole milk

1banana

1 avocado flesh (spooned out)

1 tbsp raw honey

Juice Drinks for Weight Loss

These special drinks can be taken instead of breakfast and together with balanced low calorie lunches and dinners. For faster weight loss, you may try two drinks daily plus a well balanced dinner of protein and vegetable s, total intake should not drop below 800 calories per day.

Berrylicious

2 tbsp. All vegetable High Quality protein powder

8 oz. low fat milk or orange juice

1/2 cup raspberries, boysenberries or gooseberries

Carrot Smooth

8 oz raw carrot juice

1 piece of celery

1 thick slice of green pepper

1 cored apple

Cranberry Punch

8 oz cranberry juice

2 tbsp All vegetable high quality protein powder

1 large fresh apple

Juice Drinks for Energy

These special drinks should be taken about 30 minutes prior to exercising for explosive energy. They are an excellent source of carbohydrate energy foods.

Potassium Power Punch

8 oz fresh orange juice

2 tbsp. All vegetable high quality protein powder

1 well ripened banana

Apple Crisp

8 oz. freshly juiced apples

1/2 lemon

1/2 lime

1 slice apricot, peach, mango or papaya

1/4 cup crushed ice

Power Burst

8.oz pineapple juice

1/2 pear

1/2 peach

2 tbsp. All vegetable high quality protein powder

1/4 cup crushed ice

Progress Record

Progress Record

Progress Record

Progress Record

Progress Record

Thank you for purchasing my book. I hope that you found it to be both easy to read and understandable.

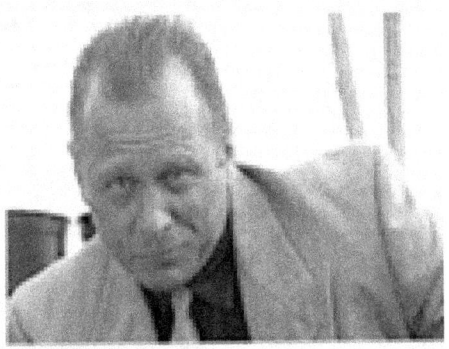

Probably no differently than anyone else I began exercising slowly and with no real knowledge of what I was getting into at all. I had no daily plan based on what I wanted to achieve and soon found myself to have more questions and concerns as every day went by. There was pain on a daily basis, there was the fear that I might be injuring myself by doing something wrong or over doing it altogether I just didn't know ...but I continued on and I soon realized, after a very short period of time that the pain and soreness would all disappear within the first 10 minutes of the next days workout, that was when I first realized that there were things going on that I didn't fully understand yet. It was that moment that I realized that the choice was mine to succeed or fail, the only question was how hard did I want it?

It wasn't long after that when I began to test the physical limits that I had placed on myself all my life, it was when I first realized that success would be on the other side of the "limit line" I've been living behind.

It was the beginning of a learning process that would span several years of my life and ultimately helped me achieve my goal of taking weight loss and muscle development to the level that I took it to and it' will help you achieve your goal as well!.

www.ingramcontent.com/pod-product-compliance
Lightning Source LLC
Chambersburg PA
CBHW060642290526
45793CB00001B/355